SOMATIC EXERCISES
for Beginners

Techniques for Nervous System Regulation, Vagus Nerve Reset, and Anxiety & Stress Relief in Under 10 Minutes a Day | 28-Day Program Included

Audrey Sweeney

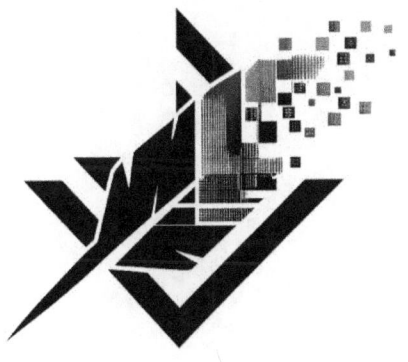

VANGUARD NOVA

© Copyright 2024 by Vanguard Nova - All rights reserved.

All rights reserved. No part of this book may be reproduced in any form without permission in writing from the author. Reviewers may quote brief passages in reviews.

While all attempts have been made to verify the information provided in this publication, neither the author nor the publisher assumes any responsibility for errors, omissions, or contrary interpretation of the subject matter herein.

The views expressed in this publication are those of the author alone and should not be taken as expert instruction or commands. The reader is responsible for his or her own actions, as well as his or her own interpretation of the material found within this publication.

Adherence to all applicable laws and regulations, including international, federal, state and local governing professional licensing, business practices, advertising, and all other aspects of doing business in the US, Canada or any other jurisdiction is the sole responsibility of the reader and consumer.

Neither the author nor the publisher assumes any responsibility or liability whatsoever on behalf of the consumer or reader of this material. Any perceived slight of any individual or organization is purely unintentional.

TABLE OF CONTENTS

INTRODUCTION — 7

The Mind-Body Connection — 9

Fundamentals of Somatic Exercises — 12

The Body's Response to Stress and Trauma — 16

Common Challenges and Solutions — 19

Creating a Safe Space for Practice — 22

FOUNDATIONAL BREATHING TECHNIQUES — 26

Exercise 1: Deep Belly Breathing — 28

Exercise 2: Alternate Nostril Breathing — 30

Exercise 3: Lengthened Exhale Breathing — 32

Exercise 4: Ocean Breath (Ujjayi) — 34

RELEASING STRESS AND ANXIETY — 36

Exercise 5: Neck and Shoulder Release — 38

Exercise 6: Gentle Twist for Tension Relief — 40

Exercise 7: Softening the Gaze (Eye Yoga) — 42

Exercise 8: Shaking and Dancing Free — 44

Exercise 9: Gentle Jaw Exercises — 46

Exercise 10: Writing for Emotional Release — 48

Exercise 11: Visualization for Calm — 50

ENHANCING SPINAL HEALTH AND POSTURE — 52

Exercise 12: Gentle Backbends — 54

Exercise 13: Supine Spinal Rotation — 56

Exercise 14: Dynamic Cobra Stretch — 58

Exercise 15: Forward Fold Series — 60

Exercise 16: Extended Puppy Pose — 62

Exercise 17: Chair Pose for Alignment — 64

Exercise 18: Downward Dog to Lengthen the Spine — 66

CULTIVATING MINDFULNESS AND PRESENCE — 68

Exercise 19: Body Awareness Meditation — 70

Exercise 20: Slow Motion Movement — 72

Exercise 21: Hand Tracing Meditation — 74

Exercise 22: Mindful Eating Practices — 76

Exercise 23: Heart-Centered Breathing — 78

PROMOTING FLEXIBILITY AND GRACE — 80

Exercise 24: Gentle Yoga Flow — 82

Exercise 25: Reclining Leg Stretch	84
Exercise 26: Dynamic Lunge Sequence	86
Exercise 27: Wrist and Ankle Rolls	88
Exercise 28: Standing Side Stretch	90
Exercise 29: Sphinx Pose for Lower Back	92
Exercise 30: Figure Four Stretch	94
Exercise 31: Restorative Hip Opening	96
Exercise 32: Gentle Neck Rolls	98
Exercise 33: Therapeutic Self-Massage Techniques	100

IMPROVING BALANCE AND MENTAL FOCUS — 102

Exercise 34: Tree Pose Variations	104
Exercise 35: Focused Gaze (Drishti) Practices	106
Exercise 36: One-Legged Balance with Arm Movements	108
Exercise 37: Stability Ball Core Focus	110
Exercise 38: BOSU Ball Balancing	112

THE BENEFITS OF VAGUS NERVE STIMULATION — 122

EXERCISES TO ACTIVATE AND TONE THE VAGUS NERVE — 124

28-DAY EXERCISE PLAN — 133

INTRODUCTION

Welcome to "Somatic Exercises For Nervous System Regulation." In this book, we embark on a journey to discover the profound connection between our bodies and our minds, and how simple yet powerful exercises can help us achieve harmony within ourselves.

Have you ever felt overwhelmed by stress, anxiety, or chronic pain? Perhaps you've experienced moments where your body feels tense and your mind races with worries. You're not alone. In today's fast-paced world, many of us grapple with these challenges, seeking relief and balance amidst the chaos of everyday life.

But fear not, for somatic exercises offer a path to tranquility and well-being. Somatic exercises focus on the body's innate wisdom, tapping into its natural ability to heal and restore equilibrium. By engaging in gentle movements, conscious breathing, and mindful awareness, we can soothe our nervous system, release tension, and cultivate a profound sense of calmness.

Throughout this book, we will delve into the principles and practices of somatic exercises, exploring their transformative potential for our physical, mental, and emotional health. Whether you're a seasoned yogi or a newcomer to mind-body practices, you'll find valuable insights and practical techniques to support you on your journey towards greater well-being.

In the following chapters, we'll unravel the mysteries of the mind-body connection, delve into the science behind somatic healing, and learn how to harness the power of our own physiology to overcome stress, trauma, and pain. We'll also explore common challenges that may arise on this path and offer guidance on how to navigate them with grace and resilience.

So, join me as we embark on this empowering journey of self-discovery and self-care. Together, we'll unlock the secrets of somatic exercises and awaken to a life of greater ease, vitality, and joy.

Let's begin our exploration into the transformative world of somatic exercises, where body and mind converge in perfect harmony.

The Mind-Body Connection

The intricate and profound connection between the mind and body is a central theme in understanding and applying somatic exercises. This connection suggests that the mind is not only housed within the body as a mere passenger but actively shapes and directs the body's health and vice versa. The mind-body connection encompasses how thoughts, feelings, beliefs, and attitudes can positively or negatively affect biological functioning, while physical states can influence mental and emotional states.

At its core, the mind-body connection is about interaction and influence. It's an acknowledgment that emotional stress can contribute to physical ailments such as hypertension, heart disease, and digestive disorders. Conversely, physical states, including posture and breathing patterns, can impact mood and stress levels. This bidirectional influence forms the foundation of somatic exercises, which utilize the body as a gateway to improve mental health and emotional well-being.

The principles behind somatic exercises are rooted in various psychological and physiological theories. One key aspect is the role of the autonomic nervous system (ANS), which regulates many organs and muscles in the body and is closely linked to our emotional state. The ANS operates largely outside of our conscious control, managing vital functions like heartbeat, breathing, and digestion. It has two main components: the sympathetic nervous system, which triggers the "fight or flight" response during perceived threats, and the parasympathetic nervous system, which promotes "rest and digest" responses. Somatic exercises aim to activate the parasympathetic system to bring about relaxation and reduce stress.

For example, controlled breathing practices, a staple in somatic exercises, directly influence the nervous system. By altering breathing patterns—slowing the breath and focusing on deep inhalations and exhalations—we can encourage the body to shift from a state of stress to one of calm. This shift is not merely subjective; it is measurable through changes in heart rate, blood pressure, and muscle tension. Such changes also feedback to the brain, signaling safety and relaxation, which helps to alleviate mental stress and anxiety.

Similarly, postural adjustments can have immediate impacts on mental states. Consider the effect of simply standing up straight with shoulders back after hours of slumping in a chair. This adjustment can increase energy levels, boost self-confidence, and improve concentration. It's a physical change that influences the psyche, demonstrating the mind-body interaction in a tangible way.

Moreover, the practice of mindfulness within somatic exercises—being fully present in the moment—enhances this connection. Mindfulness encourages an awareness of the body's sensations, the breath, and the environment, which helps to ground mental activity in the physical world. This awareness is not passive; it's an active monitoring that fosters deep understanding and management of one's thoughts and emotions, which in turn influences physical health.

The integration of mind and body through somatic exercises offers a powerful tool for health and wellness. By learning to control physiological processes and becoming more attuned to the body's signals, individuals can manage stress more effectively, improve emotional resilience, and enhance overall quality of life. This holistic approach is not just about treating or preventing illness; it's about fostering an optimal state of being where the mind and body are not merely connected, but harmoniously integrated.

Fundamentals of Somatic Exercises

Somatic exercises represent a profound and holistic approach to health and wellness, integrating the mind and body through gentle, conscious movements and breathwork. This method emphasizes internal perception and experience, focusing not just on physical movement but also on the awareness of sensations and the effects these movements have on the body and mind. Understanding the fundamentals of somatic exercises is essential for anyone looking to enhance their well-being by engaging deeply with their own body's signals and capacities.

At its heart, somatic exercises are built on the principle of soma, a Greek word meaning "living body." It is the body perceived from within, where you become deeply attuned to your own physical sensations and experiences. This internal focus is what differentiates somatic exercises from many conventional exercise routines that often prioritize external appearances or achievements.

1. **Awareness**: The first fundamental of somatic exercises is developing a heightened awareness of the body. This involves paying close attention to the feelings of movement and the subtleties of muscle tension, position, and effort. Awareness is cultivated through practices that encourage mindfulness and proprioception—the sense of the relative position of one's own parts of the body and strength of effort being employed in movement.

2. Regulation of the Autonomic Nervous System: Somatic exercises often aim to regulate the autonomic nervous system by activating the parasympathetic nervous system (PNS). The PNS is responsible for rest and digest functions, which counteract the stress response controlled by the sympathetic nervous system. Techniques such as deep diaphragmatic breathing, slow and gentle movements, and mindful relaxation are used to bring about a state of calm.

3. Movement Reeducation: Many somatic exercise systems include a form of movement reeducation where habitual patterns of movement are reexamined and often altered. This reeducation process involves unlearning maladaptive muscle patterns and learning new, more efficient, and healthier ways to move. Through this, individuals can reduce pain, improve mobility, and enhance their overall physical performance.

4. Integration: Another fundamental aspect of somatic exercises is the integration of movements into daily activities. It's not only about performing exercises in a session but also about applying the principles learned to everyday actions. This might mean adjusting how one sits, walks, or bends down to pick something up, ensuring that the body moves in a manner that is aligned and balanced.

5. Self-Regulation and Healing: Somatic exercises empower individuals to take charge of their own physiological functions. By becoming more attuned to their body's needs and responses, individuals can effectively manage stress, pain, and dysfunction on their own. This self-regulation leads to greater health autonomy and a more profound capacity for healing.

6. Holistic Health: Finally, somatic exercises approach health from a holistic perspective. Instead of treating isolated symptoms or parts of the body, this approach considers the entire person—body, mind, and spirit. It recognizes that emotional, psychological, and physical health are deeply interconnected and that addressing one aspect can lead to improvements in others.

The Body's Response to Stress and Trauma

Understanding how the body responds to stress and trauma is crucial for developing effective strategies to manage and alleviate their long-term impacts. The body's response mechanisms are sophisticated and deeply ingrained, serving essential survival functions. However, when these responses become chronic or are triggered inappropriately, they can lead to significant physical and psychological health issues.

When faced with a stressful situation or traumatic event, the body activates its autonomic nervous system (ANS), specifically the sympathetic nervous system (SNS). This activation prepares the body for rapid action—what is commonly known as the "fight or flight" response. The adrenal glands release stress hormones like cortisol and adrenaline, which trigger a cascade of physiological changes: heart rate and blood pressure increase, muscles tighten, and breathing becomes faster and shallower. This state of heightened alertness and physical readiness is essential for immediate survival but can be damaging when sustained over time.

In the short term, these responses are beneficial and necessary. They mobilize energy, enhance focus, and increase resilience, enabling an individual to cope with immediate threats. However, if the stressor is constant or the traumatic experience lingers without resolution, the body can remain in a state of high alert, leading to exhaustion and a variety of health problems.

Chronic activation of the stress response can lead to:

- **Cardiovascular issues**: Persistent increases in heart rate and blood pressure can strain the cardiovascular system, increasing the risk of heart attacks and strokes.

- **Immune system suppression**: Elevated cortisol levels can suppress the immune system, making the body more susceptible to infections and illnesses.

- **Digestive problems**: Stress can alter the gut's functioning, leading to issues like gastritis, ulcers, and irritable bowel syndrome.

- **Mental health disorders**: Prolonged stress can contribute to anxiety, depression, and post-traumatic stress disorder (PTSD).

- **Musculoskeletal disorders**: Constant muscle tension can lead to chronic pain conditions such as tension headaches, migraines, and fibromyalgia.

Beyond these direct physical effects, the body's response to stress and trauma can also alter an individual's behavior and emotions. People may experience mood swings, irritability, fatigue, difficulty concentrating, and changes in appetite or sleep patterns. These behavioral and emotional changes can further complicate the physical symptoms, creating a complex web of interrelated issues.

To manage and mitigate these responses, it is essential to engage strategies that activate the parasympathetic nervous system (PNS), the component of the ANS responsible for "rest and digest" functions. Techniques such as deep breathing, mindfulness meditation, gentle physical exercises, and somatic therapies are effective because they help the body transition from a state of stress to one of relaxation. These methods encourage the body to release tension and restore balance, promoting healing and recovery.

Moreover, understanding and recognizing the signs of stress and trauma in the body can empower individuals to take proactive steps towards self-care. Educating oneself about the body's stress responses and implementing regular practices for managing stress can prevent the escalation of symptoms and improve overall health and well-being.

Common Challenges and Solutions

Embarking on a journey of somatic exploration and healing is a courageous step towards reclaiming ownership of our bodies and minds. However, like any journey, it is not without its challenges. In this chapter, we'll explore some of the common obstacles that may arise on the path of somatic practice and offer guidance on how to navigate them with grace and resilience.

One of the first challenges we may encounter is resistance – the inner voice that whispers doubts and fears, questioning our ability to change and grow. Resistance often stems from deeply ingrained patterns of thought and behavior, rooted in our past experiences and beliefs about ourselves and the world around us. It may manifest as procrastination, self-doubt, or a reluctance to step outside our comfort zone.

But resistance is not a sign of weakness; rather, it is a natural response to the unknown and the unfamiliar. When we encounter resistance on our somatic journey, it's important to approach it with curiosity and compassion, acknowledging the underlying fears and insecurities that may be driving it. By shining a light on our resistance and befriending it with kindness, we can begin to unravel its grip and open ourselves to the possibility of growth and transformation.

Another common challenge on the path of somatic practice is discomfort – the physical sensations and emotional upheavals that arise as we engage with the deeper layers of our being. Somatic exercises have a way of stirring up dormant energies and unresolved emotions, bringing them to the surface for healing and release. While this process can be uncomfortable at times, it is also an essential part of the healing journey.

When faced with discomfort in somatic practice, it's important to remember that healing is not always linear or pain-free. Like a river carving its path through the earth, healing often involves navigating the twists and turns of our inner landscape, confronting obstacles and resistance along the way. By leaning into the discomfort with courage and compassion, we can uncover the hidden treasures that lie beneath the surface and emerge stronger and more resilient than before.

In addition to resistance and discomfort, another challenge we may encounter is doubt – the nagging voice that whispers, "Is this really working? Am I doing it right?" Doubt often arises when we're in the midst of change and uncertainty, questioning the validity of our experiences and the efficacy of our efforts. But doubt is a natural part of the human experience, reminding us to approach our journey with humility and openness.

When doubt arises in somatic practice, it's helpful to remember that healing is a gradual and iterative process, with no fixed endpoint or destination. Each step we take on the path of somatic exploration brings us closer to ourselves and the truth of our own experience. By cultivating trust in the wisdom of our bodies and the guidance of our inner teacher, we can navigate the terrain of doubt with confidence and clarity.

Creating a Safe Space for Practice

As we embark on the journey of somatic exploration and healing, it's essential to create a safe and supportive environment where we can engage with our bodies and emotions with care and compassion. In this chapter, we'll explore the importance of cultivating a safe space for somatic practice and offer practical guidance on how to create one in your own life.

A safe space is more than just a physical environment; it's a container of love, acceptance, and non-judgment where we can show up as we are, with all our strengths and vulnerabilities. Creating a safe space for somatic practice involves cultivating a sense of trust and security within ourselves and our surroundings, allowing us to relax and open to the process of healing and transformation.

One of the first steps in creating a safe space for somatic practice is to establish clear boundaries and intentions for our practice. Boundaries serve as protective barriers, delineating the space where our practice takes place and safeguarding us from external distractions and intrusions. By setting clear boundaries around our time, energy, and physical space, we create a container of safety and protection where we can immerse ourselves fully in the present moment.

In addition to boundaries, intention setting plays a crucial role in creating a safe space for somatic practice. Intentions are like guiding stars, illuminating the path ahead and orienting us towards our deepest desires and aspirations. By setting an intention for our practice – whether it's to cultivate relaxation, release tension, or deepen our connection with ourselves – we infuse our practice with purpose and meaning, anchoring ourselves in the present moment and aligning our actions with our highest values.

Another essential aspect of creating a safe space for somatic practice is to cultivate a sense of presence and mindfulness. Presence is the art of being fully engaged and attentive to the present moment, without judgment or attachment to the past or future. When we approach our practice with presence and mindfulness, we open ourselves to the fullness of our experience, allowing sensations, emotions, and thoughts to arise and pass with grace and ease.

Physical comfort is also an important consideration when creating a safe space for somatic practice. Choose a quiet, comfortable environment where you won't be disturbed, and make sure you have access to any props or equipment you may need for your practice.

Create a cozy atmosphere with soft lighting, soothing music, or aromatherapy to enhance your sense of relaxation and well-being.

Finally, remember that creating a safe space for somatic practice is an ongoing process of exploration and refinement. Be gentle with yourself and allow room for experimentation and adjustment as you discover what works best for you. Trust your intuition and listen to the wisdom of your body, honoring its needs and desires with love and compassion.

In the following chapters, we'll explore specific somatic exercises and practices to help you cultivate a deeper sense of safety and security within yourself. From breathwork and relaxation techniques to movement meditations and guided visualizations, we'll discover a wealth of resources to support you on your journey of healing and self-discovery.

FOUNDATIONAL BREATHING TECHNIQUES

Breathing is the most fundamental act of life, yet it is often overlooked as a powerful tool for health and wellbeing. In "Foundational Breathing Techniques," we explore a series of exercises that leverage the innate power of breath to regulate the nervous system, reduce stress, and enhance overall vitality.

This section is designed to introduce you to various breathing techniques that serve as the cornerstone for nervous system regulation. Each exercise in this section is meticulously chosen to help you learn how to harness the power of your breath to create profound changes in your mental, emotional, and physical states. Whether you are dealing with anxiety, seeking deeper relaxation, or simply want to improve your respiratory efficiency, these exercises provide a pathway to achieving those goals.

By practicing these techniques, you will not only improve the quality of your breath but also enhance your ability to focus, calm your mind, and respond more effectively to stress. The exercises will guide you through methods of breathing that can be used at any time and place to foster a deep sense of peace and well-being.

Exercise 1: Deep Belly Breathing

Description: Deep Belly Breathing, often referred to as abdominal breathing, is a fundamental technique for calming the nervous system. It helps switch the body from a state of stress (sympathetic nervous system activation) to a state of relaxation (parasympathetic nervous system activation). By focusing on deep, controlled breaths into the abdomen, this exercise promotes better respiratory efficiency and relaxation.

Benefits:

- Reduces feelings of anxiety and stress
- Engages the parasympathetic nervous system, promoting relaxation
- Increases the supply of oxygen to the brain and muscles
- Helps stabilize blood pressure

Steps:

1. Sit comfortably with your back straight or lie flat on a yoga mat. Place one hand on your chest and the other on your stomach.

2. Breathe in deeply through your nose, ensuring your diaphragm (not your chest) inflates with enough air to create a stretch in your lungs. Your stomach should rise, not your chest.

3. Pause for a moment at the top of your inhale, then exhale slowly and deeply through the mouth, pushing out as much air as you can while contracting your abdominal muscles.

4. Continue this pattern of breathing, focusing on the rise and fall of your abdomen, and the relaxing sensations that follow each exhale.

5. Repeat for 3-5 minutes to calm the mind and ease the body.

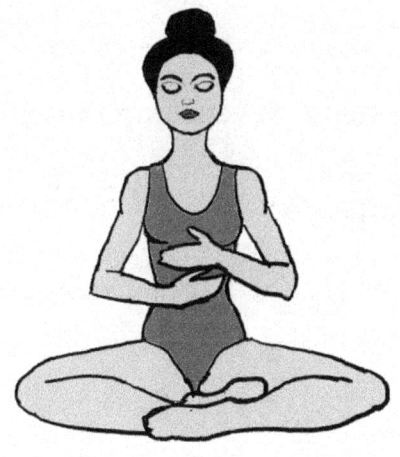

Exercise 2: Alternate Nostril Breathing

Description: Alternate Nostril Breathing, or Nadi Shodhana, is a yogic breathing technique that helps restore balance and ease in the mind and body. The practice involves alternately closing each nostril while breathing in and out. The rhythmic pattern helps harmonize the left and right hemispheres of the brain, leading to mental clarity and a calming effect on the nervous system.

Benefits:

- Enhances cardiovascular function
- Lowers stress and improves mood
- Supports lung function and respiratory endurance
- Balances the left and right hemispheres of the brain

Steps:

1. Sit in a comfortable position with a straight spine. Close your right nostril with your right thumb.
2. Inhale slowly through the left nostril, then close it with your right ring finger. Pause for a second.

3. Open the right nostril and exhale slowly through it, then inhale through the right nostril.

4. Close the right nostril with your thumb, open the left nostril, and exhale through the left nostril.

5. Continue this pattern, alternating nostrils after each inhalation, for 3-5 minutes.

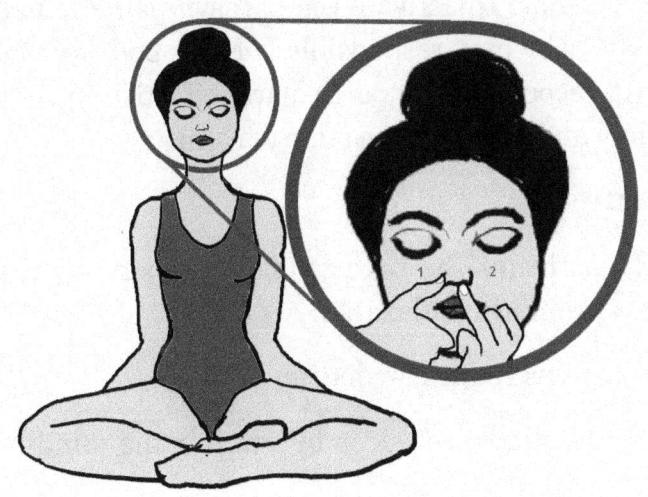

Exercise 3: Lengthened Exhale Breathing

Description: Lengthened Exhale Breathing focuses on extending the duration of the exhalation compared to the inhalation. This technique emphasizes a slower, longer exhale to activate the parasympathetic nervous system, which is responsible for the body's 'rest and digest' response. It is particularly effective in reducing anxiety and promoting a state of calm.

Benefits:

- Activates the parasympathetic nervous system, promoting relaxation
- Helps reduce anxiety and stress
- Aids in better sleep by calming the mind before bedtime
- Lowers heart rate and reduces blood pressure

Steps:

1. Find a comfortable seated position with your back straight. Close your eyes to enhance focus.
2. Inhale slowly and deeply through your nose to the count of four.

3. Exhale slowly through your mouth for a count of eight, making your exhalation twice as long as your inhalation.

4. Focus on a smooth and steady exhale, allowing all air to flow out gently.

5. Repeat this breathing pattern for 5 to 10 minutes, gradually increasing the length of the exhale as you become more comfortable with the practice.

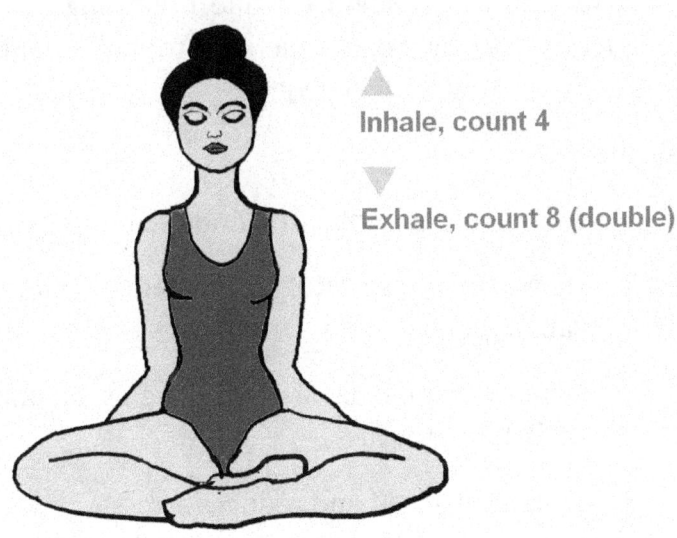

Exercise 4: Ocean Breath (Ujjayi)

Description: Ocean Breath, also known as Ujjayi Pranayama, is a classic yogic breathing technique that sounds like the gentle roar of the ocean when performed correctly. This breath is achieved by constricting the back of the throat slightly while breathing. It's used frequently during yoga practices to help focus and maintain rhythm and control.

Benefits:

- Enhances concentration and focus
- Increases respiratory efficiency and lung capacity
- Generates internal heat and helps to maintain body temperature
- Calms the mind and reduces stress

Steps:

1. Begin in a comfortable seated position with your spine erect and shoulders relaxed.
2. Inhale deeply through your nose, then constrict your throat to make a soft hissing sound like the ocean wave.

3. Keep the constriction in place as you exhale, maintaining the ocean-like sound.

4. Focus on the sound and sensation of your breathing, allowing it to be smooth and even.

5. Continue this breath for 5-10 minutes, using it to anchor your mind and steady your body's energy.

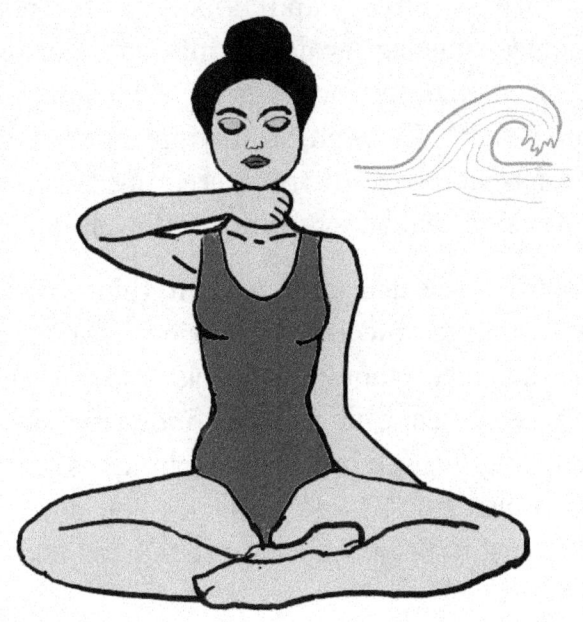

RELEASING STRESS AND ANXIETY

In this section, we focus on exercises specifically engineered to alleviate the physical manifestations of mental stress. Stress and anxiety are not just psychological states; they deeply influence our physical health, often manifesting as muscle tension, chronic pain, and fatigue. These physical symptoms can, in turn, enhance psychological distress, creating a challenging cycle of tension that affects our overall well-being.

The carefully selected exercises in this chapter are designed to target and relieve tension in critical areas such as the neck, shoulders, back, and abdomen — regions most susceptible to stress-induced discomfort. By integrating focused breathing techniques and gentle physical movements, these exercises help unravel the knots of tension, promoting a more relaxed body and a calmer mind.

Moreover, these practices are not just about physical relief; they are also deeply meditative, engaging the mind in a mindful exploration of bodily sensations. This mindful approach helps to anchor you in the present moment, effectively distancing you from stress-inducing thoughts and worries. The techniques taught here offer a dual benefit: they relax the body while simultaneously calming the mind, providing a holistic approach to stress management.

This section is designed to be practical and accessible, whether you are at home, in the office, or in any setting that allows for a few moments of self-care. Each exercise can be adapted to suit various environments and needs, ensuring that you can incorporate them into your daily routine easily and effectively.

As you work through these exercises, you'll not only learn to alleviate immediate physical discomfort but also develop strategies to manage stress more effectively in the long term. You'll gain tools that not only ease tension but also enhance your capacity to maintain calm and focus in the face of life's challenges.

Exercise 5: Neck and Shoulder Release

Description: The Neck and Shoulder Release exercise is designed to relieve tension that accumulates in the upper body, a common area where stress manifests. This exercise involves gentle stretches and mindful breathing to soften and relax the muscles around the neck and shoulders, promoting an overall sense of relaxation and ease.

Benefits:

- Relieves tension in the neck and shoulders
- Reduces headache and muscle stiffness
- Improves upper body mobility and posture
- Calms the nervous system and reduces stress

Steps:

1. Sit or stand with your spine straight and shoulders relaxed. Take a deep breath in.
2. As you exhale, gently drop your right ear towards your right shoulder, feeling a stretch on the left side of your neck.
3. Hold for a deep breath, then slowly return to the center on an inhale.

4. Repeat on the left side, dropping your left ear towards your left shoulder.

5. Perform this stretch 3 times on each side, synchronizing your movement with your breath to enhance relaxation.

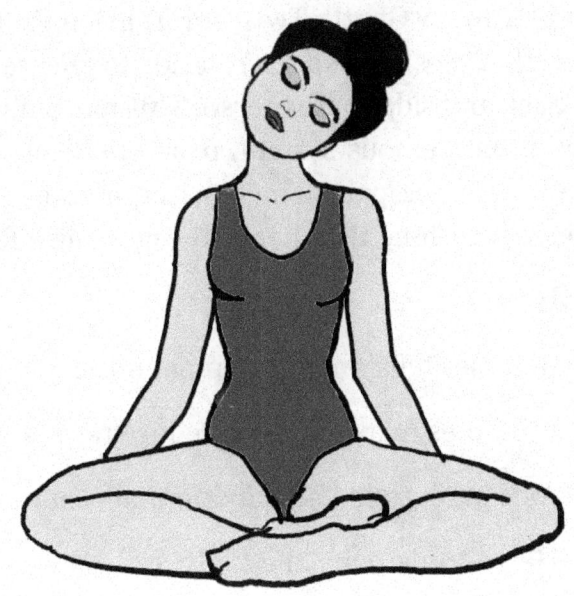

Exercise 6: Gentle Twist for Tension Relief

Description: A Gentle Twist for Tension Relief is an exercise that uses mild spinal rotation to release tension in the back and sides of the torso. This movement helps to soothe the nervous system, promote digestion, and relieve lower back pain. The twisting motion is paired with deep breathing to enhance the calming effects.

Benefits:

- Releases tension in the spinal muscles
- Promotes relaxation and reduces stress
- Aids in digestion and abdominal comfort
- Helps to detoxify the body and improve spinal health

Steps:

1. Sit on the floor with your legs crossed or in a chair with your feet flat on the ground.
2. Place your right hand behind you and your left hand on your right knee.
3. Inhale deeply, lengthening your spine upwards.

4. As you exhale, gently twist your torso to the right, looking over your right shoulder.

5. Hold this position for three deep breaths, then slowly return to the center on an inhale.

6. Repeat the twist on the left side to maintain balance in your spinal alignment.

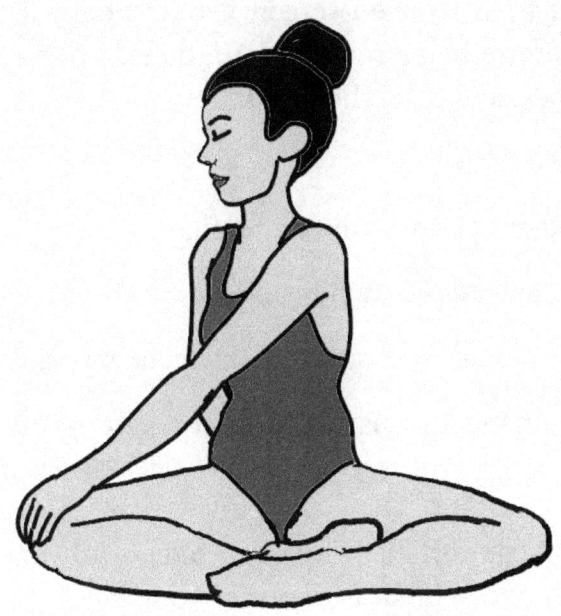

Exercise 7: Softening the Gaze (Eye Yoga)

Description: Softening the Gaze, or Eye Yoga, involves gentle eye movements and focusing techniques designed to relax the muscles around the eyes, often strained by prolonged screen use and daily stressors. This exercise helps reduce eye fatigue, soothe tension headaches, and calm the mind.

Benefits:

- Reduces eye strain and fatigue
- Alleviates tension headaches
- Promotes relaxation of the facial muscles
- Enhances focus and mental clarity

Steps:

1. Sit comfortably with a relaxed posture and take a few deep breaths to center yourself.
2. Close your eyes gently and take a moment to feel the relaxation spreading across your face.
3. Slowly move your eyeballs up and down smoothly, without straining, while keeping your eyelids closed. Repeat this movement five times.

4. Now, move your eyeballs from side to side, again with closed eyelids, repeating five times.

5. Finally, with your eyes closed, rotate your eyeballs in a full circle clockwise and then counter-clockwise, doing each direction five times.

6. Open your eyes slowly and blink a few times gently. Notice the relaxed state of your mind and eyes.

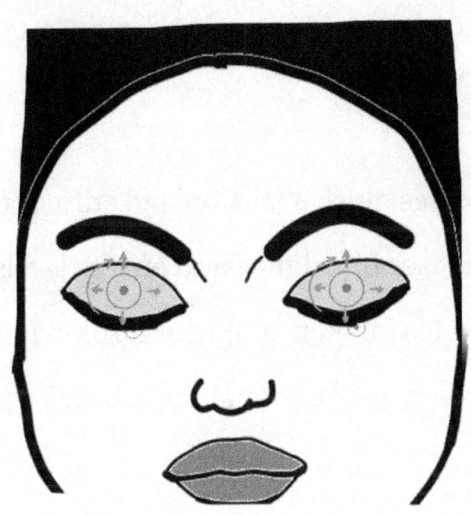

7.

Exercise 8: Shaking and Dancing Free

Description: Shaking and Dancing Free is a dynamic exercise that involves shaking your body and free-form dancing to release muscle tension and liberate pent-up energy. This practice not only loosens the physical stiffness but also boosts mood and invigorates the entire body.

Benefits:

- Releases muscle tension and stiffness
- Increases blood flow and energy levels
- Elevates mood through endorphin release
- Encourages emotional release and rejuvenation

Steps:

1. Stand with your feet hip-width apart in a comfortable space where you can move freely.
2. Begin to gently bounce on your heels, allowing your arms, shoulders, and head to shake loosely. Let your whole body vibrate as you shake off tension.

3. Gradually turn your shaking into dancing. Move however your body wants to, without thinking about rhythms or steps. Let your body lead and your mind follow.

4. Continue to dance freely for a few minutes, letting go of any rigid structures and enjoying the movement.

5. Slow down gradually and come to a standstill. Close your eyes and take deep breaths, noticing the sensations in your body and the release of energy.

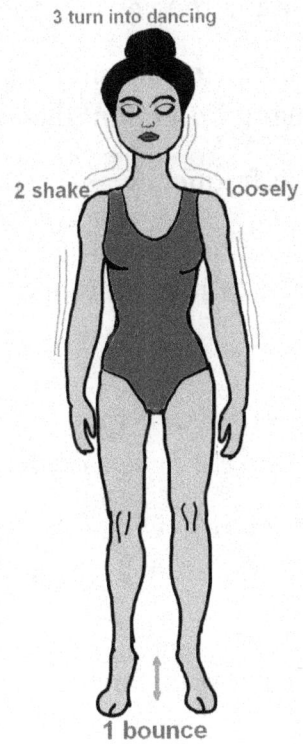

EXERCISE 9: GENTLE JAW EXERCISES

Description: Gentle Jaw Exercises focus on relieving tension in the jaw and facial muscles, areas often tight due to stress, teeth grinding, or clenching. These simple movements can help reduce discomfort, ease headaches, and promote a more relaxed state of being.

Benefits:

- Eases tension in the jaw and facial muscles
- Helps alleviate symptoms of TMJ (temporomandibular joint disorders)
- Reduces the frequency and intensity of tension headaches
- Promotes relaxation and reduces overall stress

Steps:

1. Sit or stand with your back straight and shoulders relaxed. Take a deep breath to begin.
2. Open your mouth wide, then slowly close it. Repeat this motion five times to loosen the jaw muscles.
3. Place the tips of your fingers on your jaw hinges, gently massaging in circular motions for 30 seconds.

4. Open your mouth slightly, moving your jaw side to side in a slow, controlled manner. Repeat this lateral movement five times.

5. Finally, allow your mouth to close gently. Take a deep breath in and exhale slowly, focusing on releasing any remaining tension in your jaw.

Exercise 10: Writing for Emotional Release

Description: Writing for Emotional Release is a therapeutic practice that involves expressing thoughts and emotions on paper, which can help process feelings, reduce stress, and clear the mind. This exercise facilitates a deeper connection with oneself and can lead to significant insights and emotional relief.

Benefits:

- Helps process and manage emotions effectively
- Reduces mental clutter and stress
- Enhances self-awareness and clarity
- Encourages a sense of calm and emotional balance

Steps:

1. Find a quiet, comfortable space where you can write without interruptions.
2. Choose a notebook or journal specifically for this purpose, and a pen that feels good in your hand.
3. Begin by writing down whatever comes to mind. Do not worry about grammar, spelling, or structure—let your thoughts flow freely.

4. Continue to write for at least 10 minutes, allowing yourself to explore any thoughts, feelings, or concerns that arise.

5. Once finished, you can choose to keep what you wrote, throw it away, or share it. The act of writing is where the release happens; what you do with the words afterward is up to you.

Exercise 11: Visualization for Calm

Description: Visualization for Calm is a mental exercise that involves picturing a serene and peaceful scene in your mind. This technique uses the power of the imagination to induce a state of relaxation and tranquility, helping to lower stress and improve mood.

Benefits:

- Reduces anxiety and stress
- Promotes relaxation and peace of mind
- Enhances mood and emotional resilience
- Supports better sleep quality by calming the mind before bedtime

Steps:

1. Find a quiet place where you can relax without disturbances. Sit or lie down in a comfortable position.
2. Close your eyes, take a few deep breaths, and allow your body to relax completely.
3. Picture a peaceful scene in your mind—this could be a quiet beach, a tranquil forest, or any place that you find calming.

4. Focus on the details of this scene: the sounds, the smells, the colors, and the sensations. Imagine yourself being there, feeling completely at peace.

5. Stay with this visualization for several minutes, allowing your stress to melt away as you immerse yourself in the calm of your mental oasis.

6. Gently bring yourself back to the present moment and open your eyes, carrying that sense of calm with you.

ENHANCING SPINAL HEALTH AND POSTURE

This section has introduced a variety of exercises specifically aimed at enhancing spinal health and improving posture. These exercises are designed not only to strengthen and flexibilize the spine but also to alleviate common physical ailments such as back pain and stiffness. By regularly incorporating these movements into your daily routine, you can enjoy greater mobility, reduced tension, and an overall enhanced sense of well-being.

Incorporating these practices consistently will help cultivate a healthier spine and a more balanced posture, which are essential for maintaining vitality and preventing injury as you age. Each exercise offers a unique benefit, contributing to a comprehensive approach to spinal health that supports both physical and mental health improvements.

As you progress through these exercises, observe the changes in your body's alignment, flexibility, and pain levels. Regular practice can lead to profound transformations not just physically, but also in your ability to manage stress and maintain a calm, focused state of mind.

Exercise 12: Gentle Backbends

Description: Gentle Backbends are yoga poses that stretch and open the chest, shoulders, and abdominal muscles, while also strengthening the muscles of the back and spine. This exercise improves posture, alleviates back pain, and stimulates the nervous system to enhance mood and energy levels.

Benefits:

- Enhances spinal flexibility and strength
- Opens up the chest and lungs, improving breathing capacity
- Reduces tension and pain in the lower back
- Elevates mood and boosts energy levels

Steps:

1. Start standing with your feet hip-width apart, arms by your sides.
2. Place your hands on your lower back for support, fingers pointing downward.
3. Gently arch your spine backwards, pushing your hips forward and keeping your neck in a neutral position.

4. Hold the pose for a few breaths, focusing on opening your chest and stretching your front body.

5. Slowly return to the standing position and relax your arms.

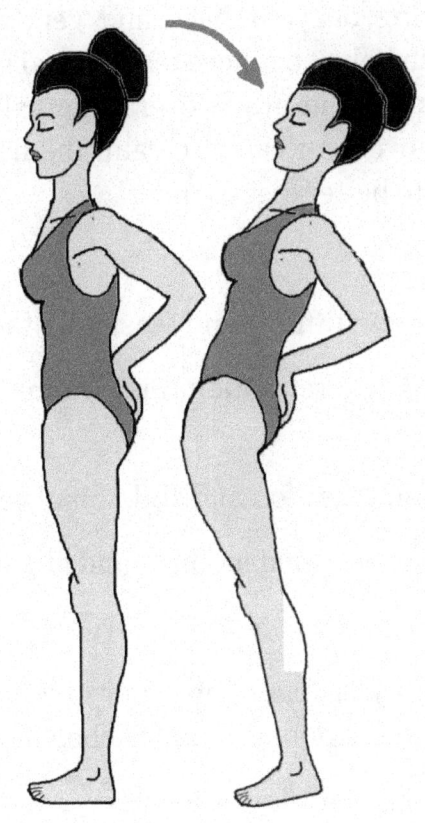

Exercise 13: Supine Spinal Rotation

Description: The Supine Spinal Rotation exercise involves lying on your back and gently rotating the spine, which helps to relieve tension and stiffness in the lower back and improve overall spinal health. This soothing movement can also calm the nervous system and promote better digestion.

Benefits:

- Relieves stiffness and tension in the spine
- Promotes relaxation and calms the nervous system
- Aids in digestion and abdominal comfort
- Improves spinal mobility and alignment

Steps:

1. Lie on your back with your knees bent and feet flat on the floor, arms stretched out to the sides.
2. Keeping your knees together, gently lower them to one side while turning your head to look in the opposite direction.
3. Hold this position for several deep breaths, allowing gravity to help deepen the stretch.

4. Slowly bring your knees back to the center and repeat on the other side.

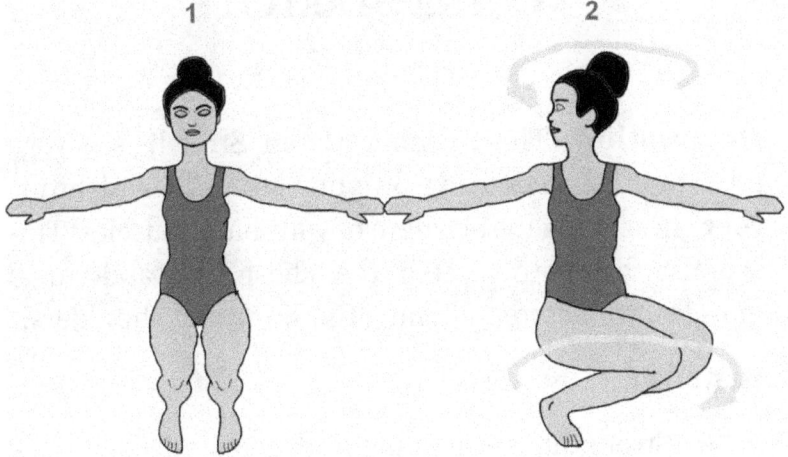

EXERCISE 14: DYNAMIC COBRA STRETCH

Description: The Dynamic Cobra Stretch is a yoga pose that involves lying on your stomach and lifting your chest using the strength of your back muscles. This exercise helps to stretch the chest and abdominal muscles, while strengthening the spine and shoulders.

Benefits:

- Strengthens the spine and helps alleviate back pain
- Opens the chest and shoulders, enhancing flexibility
- Stimulates abdominal organs, improving digestion
- Helps relieve stress and fatigue by opening the body

Steps:

1. Lie face down on the floor with your legs extended behind you and your palms placed next to your chest.
2. Press into your palms and lift your chest up, keeping your elbows slightly bent. Keep your hips and legs grounded.

3. Hold the pose for a few breaths, deepening the stretch with each exhale.

4. Slowly lower your chest back to the floor and relax.

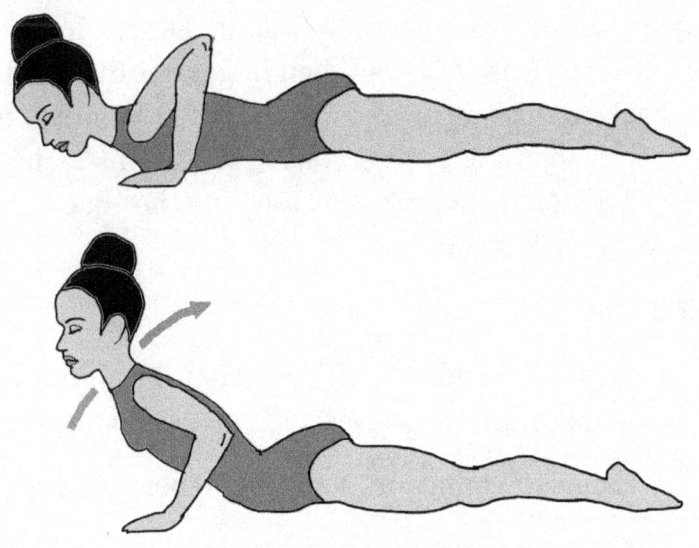

Exercise 15: Forward Fold Series

Description: The Forward Fold Series includes several variations of forward bending poses that stretch the back, hamstrings, and calves while calming the mind and soothing the nervous system. This series is beneficial for releasing tension in the back and promoting relaxation.

Benefits:

- Stretches and releases tension in the spine, hamstrings, and calves
- Calms the mind and soothes the nervous system
- Enhances flexibility in the lower body
- Promotes blood circulation to the brain

Steps:

1. Stand upright with your feet hip-width apart and your arms at your sides.
2. Inhale deeply, and as you exhale, hinge at the hips to fold forward, bending your knees slightly if needed.
3. Let your head hang loosely and your arms dangle towards the floor, or hold onto your elbows for a deeper stretch.

4. Hold this position for a few breaths, allowing gravity to pull you deeper into the stretch.

5. Gently sway from side to side if it feels comfortable, then slowly roll up to standing as you inhale.

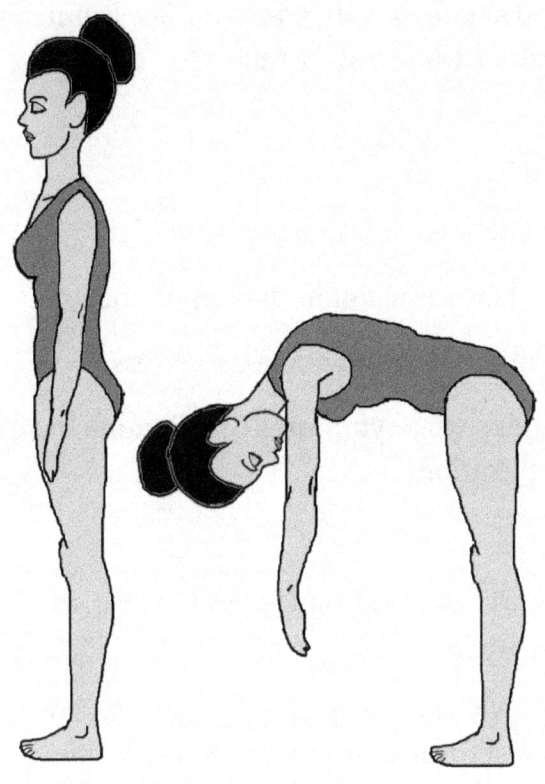

Exercise 16: Extended Puppy Pose

Description: Extended Puppy Pose is a cross between Child's Pose and Downward Facing Dog. It stretches the spine and shoulders while providing a calming effect on the mind and helping to relieve symptoms of chronic stress.

Benefits:

- Stretches the spine and shoulders
- Relieves tension in the upper body
- Calms the mind and eases stress
- Helps with symptoms of insomnia by promoting relaxation

Steps:

1. Start on your hands and knees in a tabletop position.
2. Slowly walk your hands forward, lowering your chest toward the ground while keeping your hips over your knees.
3. Extend your arms fully and rest your forehead on the floor or a block.

4. Hold the pose for a few breaths, focusing on relaxing your spine and shoulders with each exhale.

5. To release, gently walk your hands back toward your body and sit up.

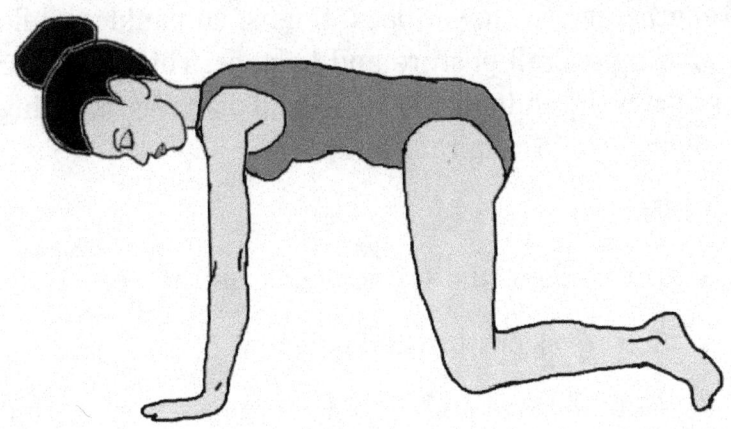

Exercise 17: Chair Pose for Alignment

Description: Chair Pose for Alignment focuses on strengthening the lower back, thighs, and ankles while improving overall posture and balance. This pose also stimulates the abdominal organs and diaphragm, aiding in digestion and respiratory function.

Benefits:

- Strengthens the spine, thighs, and ankles
- Improves posture and balance
- Stimulates abdominal organs, enhancing digestion
- Increases respiratory efficiency

Steps:

1. Stand with your feet together or hip-width apart for more stability.
2. As you inhale, raise your arms above your head, palms facing each other.
3. Exhale and bend your knees, sitting back as if you are sitting in a chair. Ensure your knees are aligned with your feet and do not extend past your toes.

4. Hold the pose for several breaths, keeping your back straight and chest lifted.

5. Inhale and straighten your legs, returning to a standing position and lowering your arms.

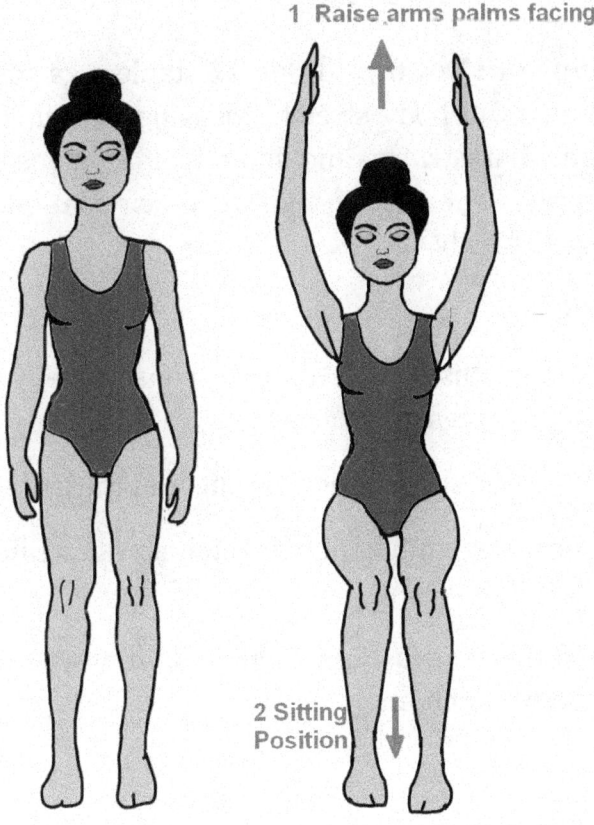

Exercise 18: Downward Dog to Lengthen the Spine

Description: Downward Dog is a staple yoga pose that serves as a full-body stretch, focusing particularly on the spine, hamstrings, and shoulders. This pose helps decompress the spine, improve circulation, and energize the body.

Benefits:

- Lengthens and strengthens the spine, hamstrings, and calves
- Enhances circulation throughout the body
- Provides a moment of inversion, which calms the nervous system
- Helps relieve back pain and improves overall body alignment

Steps:

1. Begin on your hands and knees, with your wrists aligned under your shoulders and your knees under your hips.
2. Tuck your toes under and lift your hips toward the ceiling, straightening your legs as much as

possible to form an inverted "V" shape with your body.

3. Press firmly into your hands, extending your arms and drawing your chest toward your thighs. Keep your head between your arms, aligned with your spine.

4. Hold the pose for several deep breaths, actively pushing the ground away with your hands while lifting your hips higher.

5. To exit the pose, gently lower your knees to the floor, returning to a tabletop position or sitting back into Child's Pose for a counter-stretch.

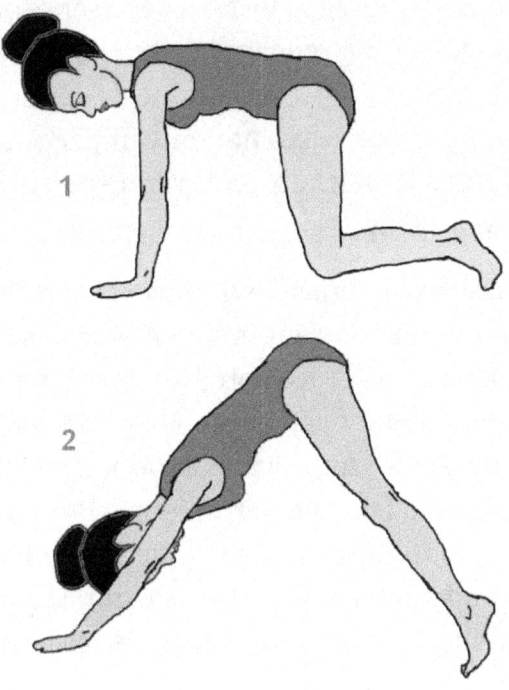

CULTIVATING MINDFULNESS AND PRESENCE

In today's fast-paced world, the ability to remain present and maintain mindfulness is more valuable than ever. Mindfulness involves a conscious effort to be aware of our experiences, thoughts, and emotions without judgment. It encourages a state of observation and reflection, helping to foster a deep sense of presence that enhances our engagement with the present moment. Cultivating mindfulness and presence through somatic exercises not only impacts mental and emotional health but also contributes significantly to physical well-being.

Mindfulness is the practice of purposely focusing your attention on the present moment—and accepting it without judgment. It is rooted in Buddhist traditions but has been popularized in the West as a powerful tool for reducing stress, improving emotional reactivity, and increasing overall cognitive resilience. Presence, closely linked to mindfulness, refers to the state of being fully engaged and attentive in the current moment, fully immersed in whatever task or experience is at hand.

Exercise 19: Body Awareness Meditation

Description: Body Awareness Meditation is a mindfulness technique that involves focusing attention on different parts of the body to enhance sensory awareness and promote relaxation. This practice helps to ground your mind in the present moment and can be particularly effective in reducing chronic stress and improving emotional regulation.

Benefits:

- Increases body awareness and sensitivity
- Helps reduce stress and anxiety
- Improves concentration and mental clarity
- Fosters a deeper sense of inner peace and calm

Steps:

1. Find a quiet place to sit or lie down comfortably. Close your eyes and take a few deep breaths to begin relaxing.
2. Start by bringing your attention to the sensations in your feet. Notice any warmth, coolness, pressure, or tingling.
3. Gradually move your focus up through each part of your body: your ankles, calves, knees, thighs,

hips, abdomen, chest, back, arms, neck, and head.

4. Spend a moment with each area, observing any sensations or lack thereof. If your mind wanders, gently bring it back to the part of the body you are focusing on.

5. Once you have moved through your entire body, take a few deep breaths, and gently open your eyes, bringing the practice to a close.

Exercise 20: Slow Motion Movement

Description: Slow Motion Movement involves performing simple physical movements at a significantly reduced speed. This exercise enhances mindfulness by requiring focused attention on every subtle movement and sensation, promoting a meditative state through motion.

Benefits:

- Enhances mental focus and mindfulness
- Reduces stress and improves mood
- Improves motor control and body awareness
- Deepens the connection between mind and body

Steps:

1. Choose a simple movement like raising your arm or walking a short distance.
2. Begin the movement very slowly, focusing on each phase of the motion as if you were moving through thick air.
3. Pay close attention to the sensations in your muscles and joints, and the feeling of your breath accompanying each movement.

4. Complete the movement and slowly reverse it, maintaining the same level of attention and slowness.

5. Repeat the movement several times, each time trying to slow down even more and deepen your focus.

Exercise 21: Hand Tracing Meditation

Description: Hand Tracing Meditation is a simple yet powerful mindfulness exercise that uses the sensory experience of tracing the hand to anchor the mind in the present moment. This technique is especially useful for those who find traditional meditation challenging, as it provides a physical focus to help maintain concentration.

Benefits:

- Promotes mental focus and reduces wandering thoughts
- Helps reduce anxiety and stress
- Enhances sensory awareness and mindfulness
- Can be used as a grounding technique during moments of overwhelm

Steps:

1. Sit in a comfortable position with your hands resting on your lap.
2. Lift one hand and, with the index finger of the opposite hand, begin to slowly trace the outline of your hand, starting from the wrist, moving up to the fingertips, and back down.

3. As you trace your hand, focus on the sensation of the skin being touched. Notice any warmth, pressure, or tingling.

4. Continue tracing your hand for several minutes, allowing your breathing to become slow and steady.

5. Once complete, repeat the process with your other hand, maintaining focus on the sensations and your breath.

Exercise 22: Mindful Eating Practices

Description: Mindful Eating Practices involve paying full attention to the experience of eating and drinking, focusing on the taste, textures, and sensations of the food. This practice helps to improve digestion, reduce overeating, and enhance your appreciation for meals.

Benefits:

- Encourages a deeper appreciation for food
- Helps regulate appetite and can aid in weight management
- Reduces digestive issues related to fast or mindless eating
- Increases satisfaction and pleasure from meals

Steps:

1. Begin by serving yourself a small amount of food in a calm environment without distractions like TV or smartphones.
2. Observe the food, noting its colors, textures, and what you imagine it will taste like.
3. Take a small bite, but do not begin chewing immediately. Notice the texture and flavors of the food in your mouth.

4. Chew slowly, being fully present with the experience of tasting and eating, noting how the flavors change.

5. Swallow mindfully, noticing the sensation of food moving down your throat.

6. Continue this process with each bite, fully engaging your senses and attention.

Exercise 23: Heart-Centered Breathing

Description: Heart-Centered Breathing focuses on directing the breath into the heart area, imagined as a way to cultivate feelings of compassion, love, and tranquility. This exercise not only reduces stress but also promotes emotional healing and connection.

Benefits:

- Fosters emotional balance and well-being
- Reduces stress and anxiety
- Enhances feelings of compassion and empathy
- Helps improve interpersonal relationships through increased emotional awareness

Steps:

1. Sit or lie down in a comfortable position and close your eyes.
2. Place your hands over your heart, feeling the rise and fall of your chest as you breathe.
3. Imagine your breath flowing in and out of your heart center, bringing warmth and light to the area.

4. With each inhale, imagine drawing in peace and calm; with each exhale, imagine releasing tension and negative emotions.

5. Continue this focused breathing for several minutes, allowing feelings of love and compassion to fill your entire being.

PROMOTING FLEXIBILITY AND GRACE

Flexibility and grace are not just physical attributes but are qualities that significantly enhance the quality of life by promoting ease of movement, reducing the risk of injuries, and maintaining a youthful vigor throughout one's life span. Somatic exercises, particularly those that enhance flexibility, are designed to nurture these qualities, allowing individuals to move with elegance and ease, regardless of their age or fitness level.

Flexibility is the ability of muscles and joints to move through their full range of motion. This capacity decreases naturally with age, but lifestyle choices, particularly levels of physical activity, significantly influence its maintenance and development. Flexibility exercises help stretch the muscles, ligaments, and tendons, which not only aids in preventing injuries but also improves posture, reduces muscle tension and soreness, and increases relaxation.

Grace in movement is often the result of not just flexibility but also strength, coordination, and balance. It involves the ability to control movements smoothly and efficiently, integrating strength with flexibility in a seamless flow. Graceful movement is not merely aesthetic; it indicates a high level of body awareness and control, which is essential for the performance of everyday activities as well as for sports and other physical pursuits.

Exercise 24: Gentle Yoga Flow

Description: Gentle Yoga Flow is a sequence of smooth, flowing yoga poses that connect breath with movement. This practice is designed to increase flexibility, reduce stress, and promote a deep sense of well-being by integrating body, mind, and spirit.

Benefits:

- Increases flexibility and muscle tone
- Reduces stress and promotes relaxation
- Enhances body awareness and coordination
- Encourages mental focus and mindfulness

Steps:

1. Start in a comfortable standing position with your feet hip-width apart, hands at your sides.
2. Inhale and raise your arms overhead, gently stretching upwards.
3. As you exhale, gracefully fold forward from the hips, hands reaching towards the ground.
4. Inhale and lift halfway up, hands on shins, back flat.

5. Exhale as you step back into a plank position, hold for a breath, then lower yourself into a low push-up.

6. Inhale as you sweep forward into an upward-facing dog, opening your chest forward and up.

7. Exhale as you push back into a downward-facing dog, holding for a few breaths.

8. Walk or step your feet back towards your hands and slowly rise to standing as you inhale, arms sweeping up.

9. Exhale and bring your hands together at heart center. Repeat the flow as desired.

Exercise 25: Reclining Leg Stretch

Description: The Reclining Leg Stretch focuses on stretching the hamstrings, calves, and lower back, which can often become tight due to prolonged sitting or standing. This exercise is performed lying down, making it an excellent choice for end-of-day relaxation.

Benefits:

- Stretches and relieves tension in the hamstrings and calves
- Reduces lower back pain and stiffness
- Improves circulation in the lower body
- Enhances flexibility and range of motion

Steps:

1. Lie on your back with both legs extended flat on the floor.
2. Lift one leg and hold the back of your thigh with both hands. If possible, straighten the leg upward, pulling gently towards your body.
3. Hold the stretch for 30 seconds to a minute, breathing deeply and focusing on relaxing the muscles.

4. Slowly release and switch to the other leg, repeating the stretch.

5. After stretching both legs, hug your knees to your chest for a gentle lower back release.

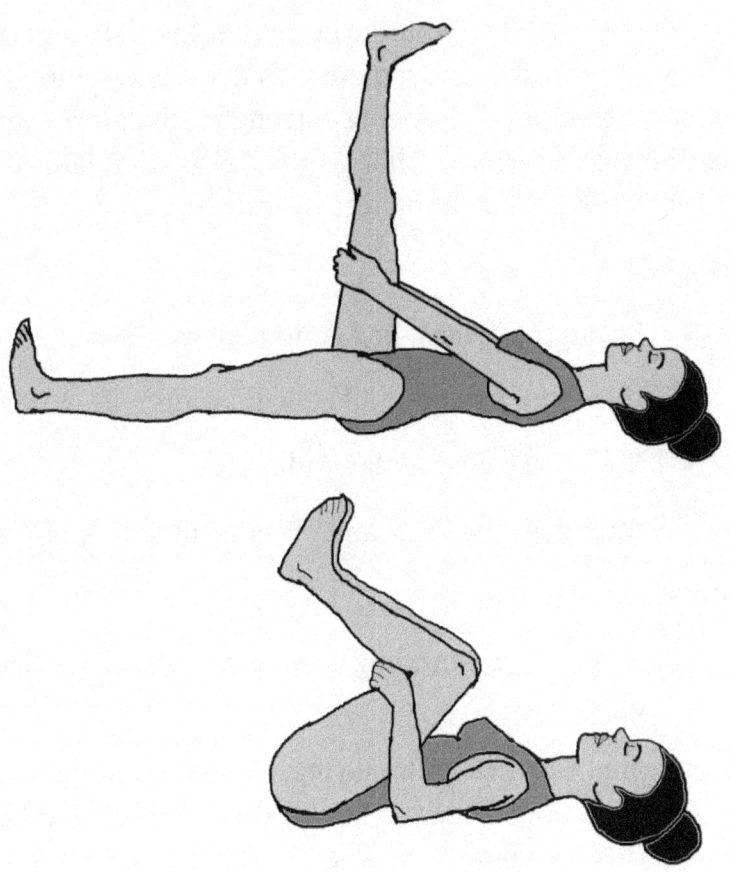

Exercise 26: Dynamic Lunge Sequence

Description: The Dynamic Lunge Sequence involves a series of lunging movements that engage multiple muscle groups, improving strength, balance, and cardiovascular health. This exercise also stimulates the nervous system and enhances overall vitality.

Benefits:

- Strengthens legs, hips, and core muscles
- Improves balance and coordination
- Boosts cardiovascular endurance
- Energizes the body and elevates mood

Steps:

1. Start in a standing position with your feet together.
2. Step forward with one leg, lowering into a lunge until both knees are bent at a 90-degree angle. Ensure your front knee is directly above your ankle.
3. Push off your front foot, returning to the starting position.
4. Repeat the lunge with the opposite leg.

5. Continue alternating legs for several repetitions, maintaining a brisk but controlled pace.

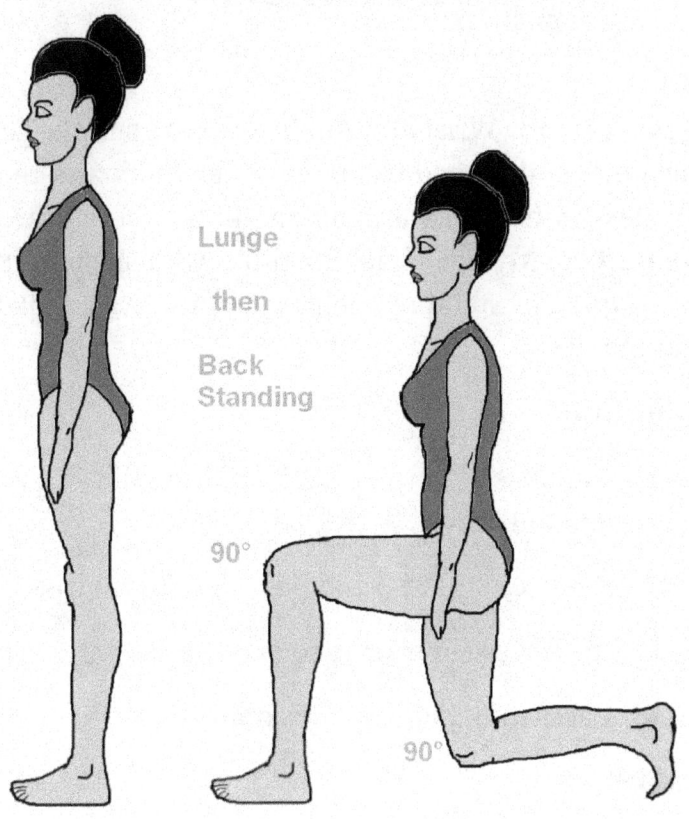

Exercise 27: Wrist and Ankle Rolls

Description: Wrist and Ankle Rolls are simple, gentle movements designed to increase flexibility and reduce stiffness in the wrist and ankle joints. These exercises are particularly beneficial for those who spend a lot of time typing or standing, helping to improve circulation and mobility.

Benefits:

- Enhances joint flexibility and mobility in wrists and ankles
- Reduces stiffness and potential for injuries
- Improves circulation to extremities
- Eases joint pain and discomfort

Steps:

1. Begin by sitting comfortably with your feet flat on the floor and your hands on your thighs.
2. Extend one arm forward, palm facing up. Slowly rotate your wrist clockwise for five rotations, then switch to counterclockwise for five rotations.
3. Repeat the same sequence with the other wrist.

4. For the ankles, extend one leg out while seated. Rotate your ankle clockwise for five rotations, then switch to counterclockwise for five rotations.

5. Repeat the ankle rolls with the other leg.

Exercise 28: Standing Side Stretch

Description: The Standing Side Stretch is an effective exercise for opening up the side body, including the ribs, hips, and lateral muscles of the abdomen. This stretch can help improve overall flexibility, enhance lung capacity, and reduce rib and back tightness.

Benefits:

- Stretches and opens the side body, enhancing lung capacity
- Improves flexibility of the spine and ribcage
- Helps alleviate pain and tightness in the lower back
- Promotes better posture and alignment

Steps:

1. Stand with your feet slightly wider than hip-width apart.
2. Raise your right arm overhead and gently lean to the left, pushing your right hip out to the side.
3. Hold the stretch for a few breaths, feeling a deep stretch along the right side of your body.

4. Return to the upright position and repeat the stretch on the left side with the left arm raised and leaning to the right.

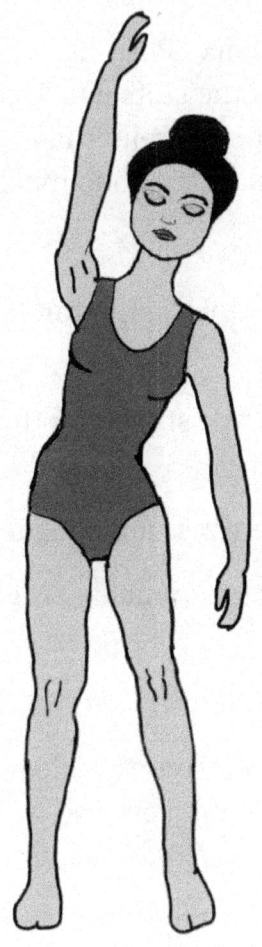

Exercise 29: Sphinx Pose for Lower Back

Description: Sphinx Pose is a gentle backbend performed lying on the stomach. This yoga pose helps strengthen the spine, rejuvenate the lower back muscles, and stimulate the abdominal organs.

Benefits:

- Strengthens the spine and tones the back muscles
- Provides a gentle stretch for the chest, shoulders, and abdomen
- Helps relieve stress and fatigue
- Stimulates abdominal organs, improving digestion

Steps:

1. Lie face down on the floor with your legs extended behind you and your elbows under your shoulders, palms facing down.
2. Gently lift your upper torso and head, engaging your lower back muscles but keeping your pelvis and legs relaxed on the floor.

3. Hold the pose for a few breaths, focusing on lengthening your spine forward and up while breathing deeply.

4. To release, slowly lower your torso back down to the floor and relax.

EXERCISE 30: FIGURE FOUR STRETCH

Description: The Figure Four Stretch is a targeted exercise that addresses tightness in the hips and glutes, areas often stressed by prolonged sitting or physical activity. This stretch can help improve flexibility, reduce hip pain, and enhance mobility in the lower body.

Benefits:

- Relieves tension and tightness in the hips and glutes
- Enhances lower body flexibility and range of motion
- Reduces pain and discomfort in the lower back and knees
- Promotes better overall posture and alignment

Steps:

1. Lie on your back with your knees bent and feet flat on the floor.
2. Place your right ankle on your left thigh just above the knee, creating a "four" shape with your legs.

3. Gently pull your left thigh towards your chest, holding the back of your thigh with both hands to deepen the stretch in your right hip.

4. Hold for 20-30 seconds, focusing on relaxing into the stretch with each breath.

5. Slowly release and switch sides, repeating the stretch with your left ankle on your right thigh.

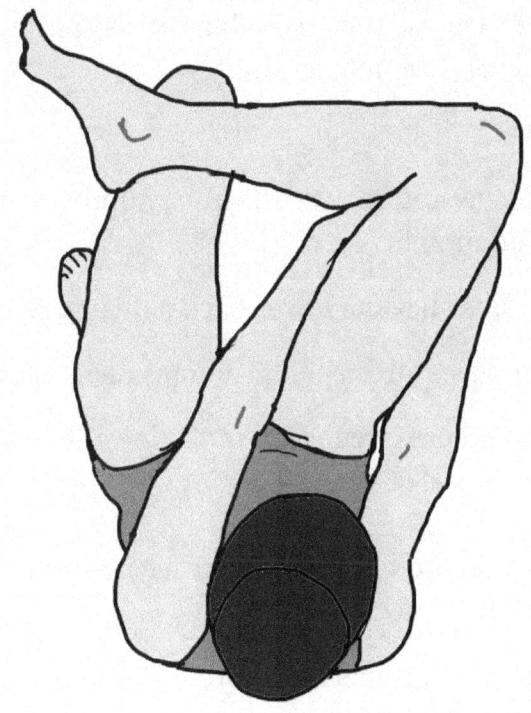

Exercise 31: Restorative Hip Opening

Description: Restorative Hip Opening involves using gentle, sustained poses to release tension in the hip area. This practice not only improves flexibility in the hips but also aids in reducing stress and anxiety by encouraging deep relaxation.

Benefits:

- Opens and relaxes the hips, improving flexibility and mobility
- Helps alleviate lower back pain and stiffness
- Reduces stress and promotes deep relaxation
- Enhances circulation in the lower body

Steps:

1. Sit on the floor with your legs extended in front of you.
2. Bend your knees and bring the soles of your feet together, letting your knees fall out to the sides.
3. Hold your feet with your hands and gently hinge forward from the hips, maintaining a straight back.

4. Hold the pose for several breaths, allowing your hips to open gradually and your body to relax deeper into the stretch.

5. To release, slowly straighten your legs and shake them gently to loosen any residual tension.

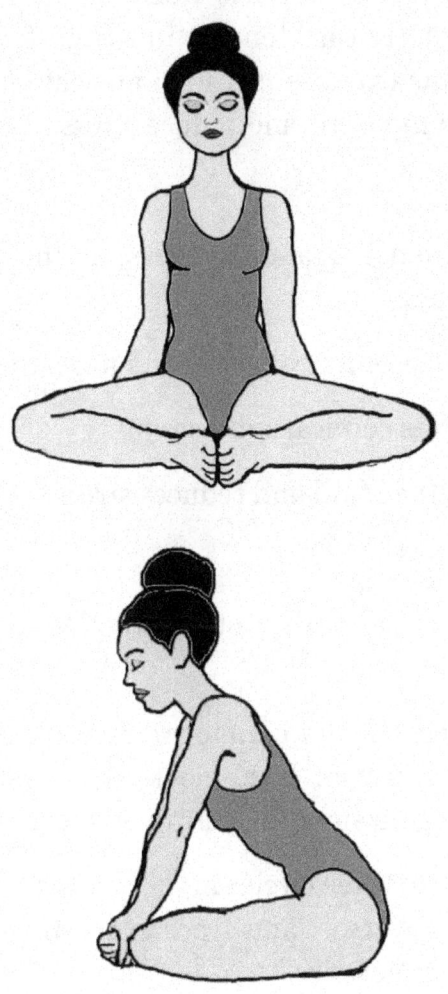

Exercise 32: Gentle Neck Rolls

Description: Gentle Neck Rolls are a simple yet effective way to release tension in the neck and upper shoulders. This exercise can help alleviate headaches, improve neck mobility, and reduce stress.

Benefits:

- Eases tension and stiffness in the neck and shoulders
- Helps prevent headaches and migraines
- Improves cervical spine mobility
- Calms the mind and reduces stress

Steps:

1. Sit or stand with a straight spine and relaxed shoulders.
2. Slowly drop your chin to your chest and begin to gently roll your head clockwise in a full circle, focusing on smooth, controlled movements.
3. Complete three circles in the clockwise direction, then reverse and perform three circles counterclockwise.

4. Keep your movements slow and deliberate, pausing if you feel any discomfort.

Exercise 33: Therapeutic Self-Massage Techniques

Description: Therapeutic Self-Massage Techniques involve using your hands to gently massage and release tension in various parts of the body. This practice can significantly improve circulation, reduce stress, and alleviate muscle soreness, providing a soothing and healing effect.

Benefits:

- Enhances circulation and stimulates lymphatic drainage
- Reduces muscle tension and soreness
- Promotes relaxation and stress relief
- Can improve sleep quality and overall well-being

Steps:

1. Choose a comfortable sitting or lying position. Use a lotion or oil if desired to reduce friction.
2. Start with your feet, using your thumbs to apply gentle pressure in circular motions, moving from your heels to your toes.

3. Work your way up to your legs, using long strokes on your calves and thighs, and circular motions around your knees.

4. Massage your hands and arms, similar to your legs, with particular attention to your wrists and forearms.

5. Use your fingertips to gently massage your neck and shoulders, employing circular motions and gentle kneading to release tightness.

6. Finish by gently massaging your scalp with your fingertips, moving in small circles across your head.

IMPROVING BALANCE AND MENTAL FOCUS

Balance and mental focus are foundational elements that support not only physical capabilities but also overall life functioning, including emotional and cognitive processes. In the realm of somatic exercises, improving balance and mental focus means engaging in practices that enhance physical stability and sharpen cognitive abilities. This integration is crucial for developing a keen awareness of the body's positioning and movements, which in turn supports higher levels of concentration and mental clarity.

Balance is a dynamic process involving the coordination of many systems within the body, including the vestibular system (inner ear balance), visual inputs, and proprioceptive feedback (sensation of body parts in space). Mental focus, on the other hand, involves the ability to concentrate one's mental effort on specific stimuli or tasks, filtering out extraneous information and distractions.

Improving balance and mental focus is particularly important as we age or engage in complex activities where precision is required.

Exercise 34: Tree Pose Variations

Description: Tree Pose Variations involve balancing on one foot while positioning the other foot on your standing leg, either on the calf or the thigh (but never on the knee). This pose helps improve balance, focus, and concentration, while also strengthening the legs and core.

Benefits:

- Improves balance and stability
- Strengthens thighs, calves, ankles, and spine
- Helps improve focus and concentration
- Encourages poise and calmness

Steps:

1. Stand tall with your arms at your sides.
2. Shift your weight to your left foot, and place the sole of your right foot on your left thigh, calf, or ankle (depending on your flexibility).
3. Once balanced, bring your hands together in prayer position at your chest, or raise them above your head.

4. Hold the pose for 30 seconds to 1 minute, maintaining steady breathing.

5. Gently lower your arms and leg and switch sides.

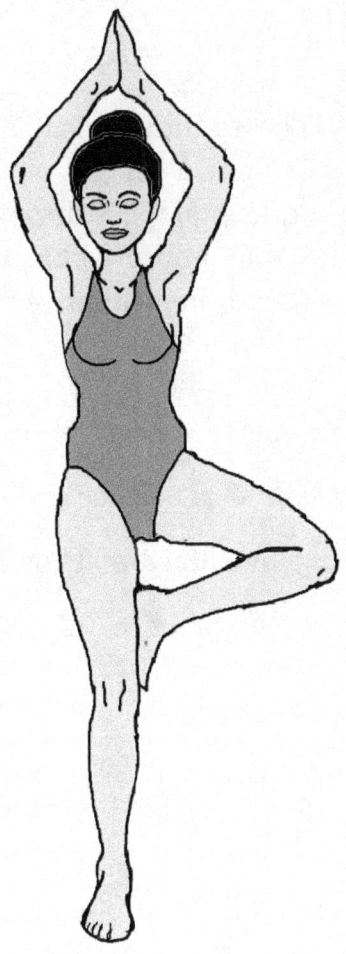

Exercise 35: Focused Gaze (Drishti) Practices

Description: Focused Gaze (Drishti) Practices involve fixing your gaze on a single point to enhance concentration and mental focus during physical poses. This practice not only improves balance and physical alignment but also aids in meditative focus.

Benefits:

- Enhances mental concentration and focus
- Improves physical balance and stability
- Promotes a meditative state of mind
- Deepens the practice of mindfulness and presence

Steps:

1. Choose a comfortable standing or seated position.
2. Select a point in front of you that is stationary. Softly focus your gaze on this point.
3. Maintain this focused gaze as you breathe deeply and evenly, keeping your body still.

4. Hold your gaze for 2-3 minutes, allowing your mind to clear and your attention to sharpen.

5. Gently relax your gaze and close your eyes for a moment to reflect on the experience.

Exercise 36: One-Legged Balance with Arm Movements

Description: One-Legged Balance with Arm Movements combines the challenge of standing on one leg with the dynamic motion of the arms, which adds a layer of difficulty and helps improve coordination and mental focus.

Benefits:

- Enhances overall balance and stability
- Improves coordination and motor skills
- Strengthens leg muscles and core
- Increases concentration and mental focus

Steps:

1. Stand tall with your feet together and arms at your sides.

2. Shift your weight onto your right foot and slowly lift your left foot off the ground, bending the knee to bring the foot up towards the buttocks.

3. Once stable, extend your arms out to the sides at shoulder height.

4. Slowly move your arms in small circles while maintaining your balance. Continue for 30 seconds.

5. Lower your arms and leg, then switch to the other leg and repeat the exercise.

Exercise 37: Stability Ball Core Focus

Description: The Stability Ball Core Focus exercise utilizes a stability ball to challenge the core muscles while maintaining balance. This exercise not only strengthens the core but also enhances focus as you work to stay balanced on the unstable surface.

Benefits:

- Strengthens the core muscles, improving posture and balance
- Enhances focus and concentration
- Engages multiple muscle groups for overall body conditioning
- Develops proprioception and body awareness

Steps:

1. Sit on a stability ball with your feet flat on the floor, hip-width apart.
2. Place your hands behind your head or across your chest.
3. Engage your core and slowly lean back slightly, then return to the upright position. Maintain your balance on the ball throughout the movement.

4. For added challenge, lift one foot off the floor while performing the leans. Alternate feet with each set.

5. Perform 10-15 repetitions, focusing on maintaining a tight core and steady breathing.

Exercise 38: BOSU Ball Balancing

Description: BOSU Ball Balancing involves using a BOSU ball—a fitness training device that looks like a stability ball cut in half with a flat platform. This exercise challenges your balance and stability by requiring you to maintain equilibrium on the unstable, dome-shaped surface, which activates core muscles and improves focus.

Benefits:

- Enhances balance and stability
- Strengthens core muscles, improving overall posture
- Increases foot, ankle, and leg strength
- Sharpens mental focus and concentration

Steps:

1. Place the BOSU ball dome-side up on a stable surface.
2. Carefully step onto the BOSU ball, starting with one foot and then the other, until you are standing in the center of the dome.

3. Once balanced, slowly shift your weight from side to side and front to back to engage different muscle groups.

4. Try to maintain your balance for 1-2 minutes, focusing on keeping your core tight and your body upright.

5. For an added challenge, perform squats, lift one leg at a time, or even close your eyes briefly to further test and improve your balance.

HARNESSING THE HEALING POWER OF THE VAGUS NERVE

The vagus nerve, derived from the Latin word for "wandering," is aptly named for its extensive reach throughout the human body. It is the longest cranial nerve, extending from the brainstem down to the abdomen, and it touches virtually every organ along the way. This section will delve into the anatomy of the vagus nerve, its crucial functions, and its impact on both physical and mental health.

Anatomy of the Vagus Nerve The vagus nerve begins at the base of the brain and wanders throughout the body, branching out to the tongue, pharynx, vocal cords, lungs, heart, stomach, and intestines. This widespread network allows it to perform a myriad of functions, acting as the command center for the parasympathetic nervous system—often referred to as the "rest and digest" system.

Functions of the Vagus Nerve The primary role of the vagus nerve is to mediate nerve impulses to and from the brain, heart, lungs, and digestive tract. It is instrumental in regulating heart rate, gastrointestinal peristalsis, sweating, and muscle movements in the mouth, including speech, swallowing, and the gag reflex. Moreover, it plays a critical role in reducing inflammation by releasing anti-inflammatory substances.

Impact on Health The health of the vagus nerve is crucial for overall well-being. It influences:

- **Heart Health:** It helps to control heart rate and blood pressure, reducing the risk of heart disease.

- **Digestion:** It stimulates the muscles in the stomach to contract and relax, promoting digestion.

- **Mood Regulation:** It affects your mood and stress levels through its interaction with certain brain regions. High vagal tone (the ability of the vagus nerve to activate quickly) is associated with a greater ability to relax after stress.

Vagal Tone and Its Importance Vagal tone is an indicator of the health of the nervous system. Individuals with a high vagal tone can relax more quickly after stress, which is reflected in their ability to regulate blood glucose levels, reduce inflammation, and even manage psychological well-being. Conversely, a low vagal tone is often associated with inflammation, negative moods, loneliness, and heart attacks.

Dysfunction of the Vagus Nerve When the vagus nerve is not functioning properly, it can lead to a range of issues, including:

- **Digestive Disorders:** Poor vagus nerve function can result in slow digestion, constipation, and nutrient absorption issues.

- **Mood Disorders:** Reduced vagal tone is observed in various conditions, including depression and anxiety.

- **Chronic Inflammation:** Inadequate regulation of the inflammatory response, potentially leading to multiple chronic illnesses.

THE BENEFITS OF VAGUS NERVE STIMULATION

Stimulating the vagus nerve can have profound effects on your body and mind, enhancing your ability to manage stress, reduce anxiety, and maintain physical health. This section explores the significant benefits of vagus nerve stimulation, with a focus on its impact on mental health, physical health, and overall emotional resilience.

Enhanced Mental Health

1. **Reduced Anxiety and Stress**: Regular stimulation of the vagus nerve helps lower the body's stress responses, reducing symptoms of anxiety and stress. By activating the parasympathetic nervous system, it encourages a state of calm and relaxation, allowing you to recover more quickly from stress-inducing situations.

2. **Mood Improvement**: The vagus nerve has direct connections to areas of the brain that regulate mood and emotions. Activating this nerve can increase the release of mood-enhancing neurotransmitters, such as serotonin and dopamine, which can help alleviate symptoms of depression.

Improved Physical Health

1. **Heart Health**: Vagus nerve stimulation has been shown to lower heart rate and blood pressure, reducing the strain on the heart and decreasing the risk of heart-related illnesses.

2. **Digestive Function**: Because the vagus nerve controls the movement and function of many parts of the digestive system, stimulating it can improve gut motility and secretion, leading to better digestion and absorption of nutrients.

3. **Reduced Inflammation**: The vagus nerve can regulate the body's immune response and reduce inflammation by releasing acetylcholine, a

neurotransmitter that acts as an anti-inflammatory agent. This is particularly beneficial for managing chronic conditions like arthritis, cardiovascular diseases, and bowel disorders.

Emotional Resilience

1. **Stress Recovery**: By improving vagal tone through regular stimulation, individuals can enhance their ability to shift more rapidly from a state of stress to relaxation, increasing resilience to daily stressors.

2. **Enhanced Connection and Social Engagement**: The vagus nerve affects communication by controlling muscles in the throat and face, essential for expressing emotions and engaging in social interactions. Improved vagal tone can lead to better emotional expressions and social connections, which are vital for emotional health.

3. **Mind-Body Connection**: Regular activation of the vagus nerve helps heighten body awareness—a key

component of mindfulness, which has been shown to improve mental health outcomes. This greater connection between mind and body can lead to an enhanced sense of control over physiological and psychological states, empowering individuals to manage their emotions and reactions effectively.

EXERCISES TO ACTIVATE AND TONE THE VAGUS NERVE

This section introduces a variety of practical exercises specifically designed to stimulate the vagus nerve. Each technique is easy to implement, taking less than 10 minutes a day, and will help you activate your body's natural relaxation response, reduce anxiety, and manage stress more effectively. Among these techniques, the king of the vagus nerve exercises is featured in a special video, which you can easily access to enhance your practice.

To watch the video, simply follow this 3-step guide:

1. **Locate the QR Code**: Find the QR code printed below or at the end of this section in your book.
2. **Scan the QR Code**: Use your smartphone's camera or a QR code

scanner app to scan the code. Point your camera steadily at the code until it recognizes and prompts you.

3. **Watch the Video**: Once scanned, a notification will appear on your screen. Tap this notification to be directed to the video. The video is downloadable and can be viewed directly on your device, allowing you to watch and follow along with the exercise anytime and anywhere.

1. **Humming**
    - **Exercise Description**: Humming naturally stimulates the vagus nerve because it causes vibrations in the body that activate this nerve.
    - **Steps to Perform**: Sit comfortably or lie down. Begin to hum a single tone and feel the vibrations along your throat and chest.
    - **Vagus Nerve Activation through Sound Vibration**: The vibrations help to increase vagal tone and promote relaxation.
2. **Gargling**
    - **Exercise Description**: Gargling with water is a simple way to stimulate the vagus nerve, which is connected to the muscles in the back of the throat.
    - **Steps to Perform**: Fill your mouth with water, tilt your head

back, and gargle the water for about 30 seconds, then spit it out.

- **Impact on Vagus Nerve through Throat Muscles**: Activates the vagus nerve by engaging the muscles at the back of the throat.

3. **Cold Water Face Splash**

    - **Exercise Description**: Cold water on your face stimulates the vagus nerve by activating the body's dive reflex, which helps to lower heart rate and blood pressure.

    - **Steps to Perform**: Splash cold water on your face several times, particularly focusing on the area beneath your eyes and above your cheekbones.

    - **Reflex Stimulation of the Vagus Nerve**: Triggers a parasympathetic response, calming the body down.

4. **Singing or Chanting**

    - **Exercise Description**: Like humming, singing and chanting can stimulate the vagus nerve due to the vibrations in the vocal cords.

    - **Steps to Perform**: Choose a song or chant and sing or chant it in a comfortable, resonant tone.

    - **Emotional and Physiological Benefits**: Enhances vagal tone and reduces stress through vocal vibration.

5. **Foot Massage**

    - **Exercise Description**: Massaging the feet can activate vagus nerve endings that are linked to various body parts, promoting relaxation.

    - **Steps to Perform**: Use firm pressure to massage the bottom of your feet, focusing on the center just below the balls of your feet.

- **Reflexology Points for Vagus Nerve Stimulation**: Stimulates areas connected to the vagus nerve, promoting relaxation.

6. **Legs Up the Wall Pose**

    - **Exercise Description**: This restorative pose helps to calm the nervous system and is effective in stimulating the vagus nerve.

    - **Steps to Perform**: Lie on your back and extend your legs up against a wall. Keep your arms by your sides and breathe deeply.

    - **Enhanced Vagal Tone and Relaxation**: Helps in blood flow regulation and activates the vagus nerve.

7. **Slow and Gentle Neck Stretches**

    - **Exercise Description**: Gentle neck stretches can stimulate the vagus nerve fibers running through the neck area.

- **Steps to Perform**: Rotate your neck slowly in a circular motion, and then gently stretch your neck from side to side.

- **Direct Stimulation of Vagus Nerve Pathways in the Neck**: Increases blood flow and activates the nerve.

8. **Deep Relaxation Meditation**

    - **Exercise Description**: Deep relaxation meditation techniques can profoundly impact vagal tone by reducing stress and promoting a state of calm.

    - **Steps to Perform**: Sit in a quiet and comfortable place, close your eyes, and focus on deep, slow breathing, envisioning your body releasing tension with each exhale.

    - **Inducing a Parasympathetic State through Mindful Breathing**: Enhances the body's relaxation response and stimulates the vagus nerve.

9. **Laughter Therapy**

    - **Exercise Description**: Laughter naturally stimulates the vagus nerve due to the rhythmic contraction of the diaphragm and other parts of the respiratory system.

    - **Steps to Perform**: Watch funny videos, join a laughter yoga class, or simply share jokes with friends. Aim to incorporate genuine laughter into your daily routine.

    - **Benefits**: Laughter triggers a relaxation response, enhancing vagal tone and reducing stress hormones in the body.

10. **Probiotic Intake**

    - **Exercise Description**: The gut-brain axis is significantly influenced by the vagus nerve, and a healthy gut can positively impact vagal tone.

    - **Steps to Perform**: Incorporate probiotic-rich foods like yogurt, kefir, sauerkraut, and other fermented foods into your diet.

- **Impact on the Vagus Nerve**: Enhances gut health, which in turn positively affects the vagus nerve by sending beneficial signals to the brain, thus promoting an overall sense of calmness.

11. **Guided Slow Breathing**

    - **Exercise Description**: Slow breathing exercises can directly stimulate the vagus nerve by reducing the heart rate and promoting relaxation.

    - **Steps to Perform**: Use a guided breathing app or timer to practice slow breathing techniques, such as inhaling for a count of four, holding for a count of seven, and exhaling for a count of eight.

    - **Vagus Nerve Activation**: This practice increases parasympathetic activity and improves heart rate variability, a key indicator of vagal tone.

12. **Tai Chi**

- **Exercise Description**: Tai Chi, a form of gentle martial arts, involves slow, deliberate movements and deep breathing, which enhance vagal activation.

- **Steps to Perform**: Join a Tai Chi class or follow an online video tutorial to learn the basic movements. Focus on the fluidity of the motions and synchronizing them with your breathing.

- **Holistic Benefits**: Tai Chi not only stimulates the vagus nerve but also improves balance, flexibility, and mental focus, contributing to reduced stress and anxiety levels.

30-DAY SOMATIC EXERCISE PLAN

Week 1: Foundation of Breath

- **Day 1: Deep Belly Breathing** - Practice for 10 minutes, focusing on deep, slow inhales and exhales.

- **Day 2: Alternate Nostril Breathing** - Alternate breathing through each nostril for 10 minutes to balance the body.

- **Day 3: Lengthened Exhale Breathing** - Spend 10 minutes practicing exhales that are twice as long as inhales.

- **Day 4: Ocean Breath (Ujjayi)** - Perform Ujjayi breathing for 10 minutes, focusing on the sound of the breath.

- **Day 5: Review Day** - Practice each breathing technique for 2 minutes.

- **Day 6: Neck and Shoulder Release** - Perform gentle stretches to release tension for 10 minutes.

- **Day 7: Gentle Twist for Tension Relief** - Do seated or standing gentle twists for 10 minutes.

Week 2: Releasing Stress and Anxiety

- **Day 8: Softening the Gaze (Eye Yoga)** - Practice eye movements and focus adjustments for 10 minutes.
- **Day 9: Shaking and Dancing Free** - Shake off tension and dance freely for 10 minutes.
- **Day 10: Gentle Jaw Exercises** - Perform exercises to release jaw tension for 10 minutes.
- **Day 11: Writing for Emotional Release** - Spend 10 minutes writing out thoughts and feelings.
- **Day 12: Visualization for Calm** - Engage in guided visualization for relaxation for 10 minutes.
- **Day 13: Review Day** - Revisit any exercises from the week that felt particularly beneficial.
- **Day 14: Rest Day** - Take a gentle walk, focusing on deep breathing.

Week 3: Enhancing Spinal Health and Posture

- **Day 15: Gentle Backbends** - Practice gentle backbends for 10 minutes.
- **Day 16: Supine Spinal Rotation** - Perform gentle twists lying on your back for 10 minutes.
- **Day 17: Dynamic Cobra Stretch** - Do gentle cobra stretches to strengthen the spine for 10 minutes.

- **Day 18: Forward Fold Series** - Engage in a series of gentle forward folds for 10 minutes.

- **Day 19: Extended Puppy Pose** - Hold the puppy pose for a total of 10 minutes, with breaks.

- **Day 20: Chair Pose for Alignment** - Perform chair pose intermittently for 10 minutes.

- **Day 21: Review Day** - Focus on spinal exercises that provided the most relief.

Last Week: Mindfulness and Flexibility

- **Day 22: Body Awareness Meditation** - Meditate with focus on body sensations for 10 minutes.

- **Day 23: Slow Motion Movement** - Practice moving in slow motion, focusing on each movement for 10 minutes.

- **Day 24: Hand Tracing Meditation** - Trace your hands slowly and mindfully for 10 minutes.

- **Day 25: Mindful Eating Practices** - Eat a meal mindfully, focusing on each bite for at least 10 minutes.

- **Day 26: Heart-Centered Breathing** - Focus on breathing into the heart space for 10 minutes.

- **Day 27: Gentle Yoga Flow** - Engage in a simple yoga flow sequence for flexibility for 10 minutes.

- **Day 28: Review Day** - Choose your favorite mindfulness or flexibility exercises and practice for 10 minutes.

www.ingramcontent.com/pod-product-compliance
Lightning Source LLC
Chambersburg PA
CBHW070251230526
45470CB00002B/562